MOTHERHOOD IS THE GREATEST THING AND THE HARDEST THING

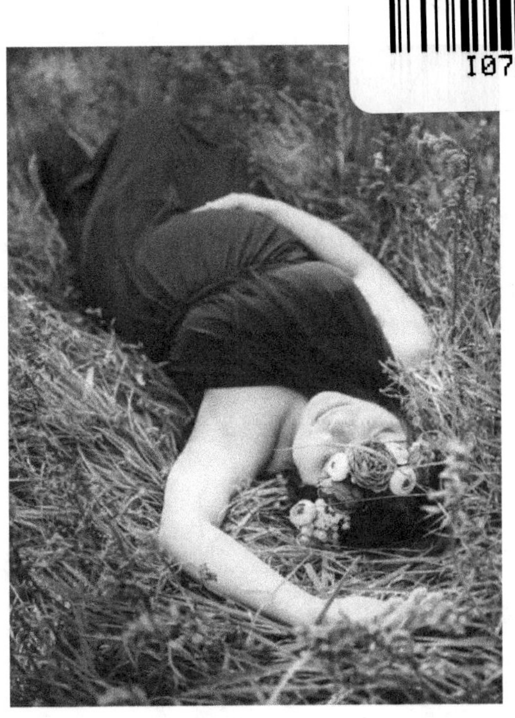

Cristina Olsen

MOTHER'S FIRST PREGNANCY

The best gift for women is the gift of Motherhood for the First time.

All of you absolutely need to get prepared for childbirth and find out what awaits you next...

TABLE OF CONTENTS

INTRODUCTION

Being pregnant comes with a lot of emotions that you never realized you had!

Are you becoming a mother for the first time?

Do you want to become worthy of the role?

If yes, keep reading!

The transformation of coming to be a mother is so fascinating that a woman shirks the entire world and considers herself as the fortunate damsel who has been given recourse to birth a child. This imagination is so full of love, affection, and devotion for the upcoming little angel, and the mother gets prepared for the mission for her whole existence. Hence, life is replenished with obstacles and impediments, and hence, the woman is the lucky gender who earns God's blessing having an alluring repercussion, feeling the strength of empowering the whole world.

However, the first pregnancy of the woman is a totally unusual concern and persists with a surplus of undertakings for you. Moreover, these tasks start from day one after the analysis of your embryo.

Congratulations! You are going to be a mother.

This was the beautiful utterance that embarked in my ears, and my heart pounded with joy and pleasure; I felt it would jump out of my chest. Retaining enthusiasm, I started plotting for the upcoming 36 weeks, and the prominent blunder I worked out was to listen on everyone's proposals and recommendations, heed their ordeals, strived to pursue their antidotes and a part of all this. I furthermore squandered my endurance in scanning assortments of editions, scrolled hundreds of Facebook pages, and searched through Google for each and every aspect. This was me during the first term of my pregnancy, and I wished to comprehend even a single tip of proficiency for giving birth to a child, but unfortunately, all this drill made me confused about what to follow and what to avoid, which I came to realize when the opportunity had ratified from my hands.

Intention of manuscript

I feel the same sentimental wing in other ladies who are going to be mothers. Certainly, each procedure has distinct viewpoints, which altogether make the whole scenario fussy and put out a disturbing situation for the pregnant one. So I determined to compile extensively valuable data for the candid mommies and intend to offer you the promising suggestion for how to steer the first pregnancy interval in satisfied orientations.

In the radiance of this catalog, you will be cognizant of the pre-birth and post-birth tactics, and you can enrich the phases of your pregnancy. Following this book, the information will surely not confront you with complications throughout the duration.

"The first Mother's Pregnancy" is the Bible for future mothers giving birth to a tot. It is a widespread but extraordinary assignment for the women. But obviously, not everyone's predicament is similar; each woman's outbreak is varied from others, so don't fritter your energy in applying other's do's and don'ts. Do your own thing with having precise guidance.

I want you to be educated on your gross duration's ups and downs, so no need to panic with the disruption promised throughout your pregnancy because this book will deliver you strength and vitality to monitor your symptoms and contour yourself. Moreover, it assembles the instant therapy of your worries and woes during your pregnancy challenges. Now, do not dehydrate with a lot of research and exploration.

Let's drive further with this week-to-week and

month-to-month instructor encompassing the pointers to spend critical milestones with a susceptible and positive set of advice for an expecting woman.

CHAPTER 1
OVERVIEW FOR 1ST TRIMESTER

Welcome to the indispensable ally with which you will discover that the next nine months and the following ones will be the most beautiful of your life.

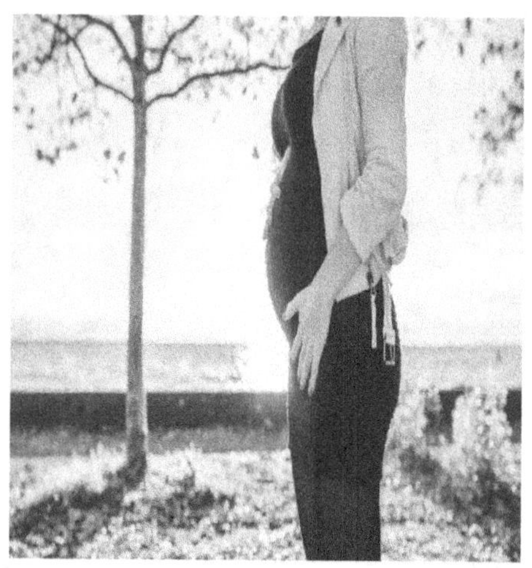

Mostly, the primary incubation is noticed in the initial month, some women compose a home trial using the pregnancy test strip, and in these days, you try to decipher about your infusions and movements.

Being a mother for the first time does not mean following already written rules that often induce anxiety. I don't teach at school, and I don't have the inherent, but I can help you with my experiences.

This step is called 1st trimester, and there would be some psychological and hormonal modifications seen in the body. These alterations do not look favorable, but they worth their existence without preference. The most ordinary of them are

- Mood swings

- Lack of appetite

- Drowsiness

- Excess of heartbeat

- Nausea

- The body twitches especially legs

- Breathing changes

- Slight pain in the lower abdomen

- Heartburn, etc.

So when you get pregnant, be watchful for all those effects that will rapidly influence your personal life and indirectly pertained to your family.

✕ You cannot eliminate these abrupt changes, but you can underrate their consequences by using your intelligence.

First, try to control your vomits because this is the way that promptly offends the neonate's existence. Due to consistent squeamishness, you can be dehydrated, which is not good for your health. If you don't like to take water solely, you can consume fresh fruit juices and fluids. This will minimize your vomiting, and you will be able to conserve yours and your fetus's vigor. Afterward, your body switches to drowsiness due to the depressed blood pressure, which will result in rigid vomits.

The next critical virtue is the swinging of your attitude because of your incredible natural adaptation; you may start feeling irritable and abhor the same stuff which you prefer largely in normal life.

These days you crave to conspire the elements that you prefer to accomplish. After the analysis, endeavor to use up your moments in these actions, which makes you become happier.

In this interval, you might suffer from active heartbeat, lack of inhaling, legs and thighs kinks, abdominal discomfort and many other trivial situations but memorize this; instead of fearing you should try some stand-ins for example after committing practiced chores and performing your obligations you should take consolation because, in this stage, you are not allowed to take even ordinary medicines for the sake of the new one's existence. You can only use medically prescribed vomiting pills before holding a meal. However, pregnancy is not an ailment, so no need to put up with superfluous nap, but in the first trimester, you can seize a little more rest due to these miseries which you are withstanding in the start. It is nice to assure you that all these physical drawbacks are limited to the first trimester.

Now, the next movement you should conduct is to carry the medical assistance in between the 6th and 7th weeks of incubation for the timely supervision of you and the baby's fitness.

Be adept! You are now getting on to inquire from the practitioner for the following sections :

- When did your last menstrual cycle show up?

- What was the aforementioned treatment or the procedure of drugs you have carried?

- How do you feel nowadays?

- You and your family's medical record

- Any genetic or chromosomal ailment or any birth structural depletion in you, your husband, or in the paternal and maternal of the unborn baby.

Afterward, you will go through the diagnosis and the screening procedure in which blood and urine examination are conducted. The third month of pregnancy indicates that the infant's body system is structured and the heartbeat transpires. So you would be examined with an ultrasound of pelvic to see the delinquent growth figuratively.

After your complete checkup, you are prescribed for some medical supplements like calcium, vitamin C, vitamin B, folic acids, etc. These medicines provide you an additional fuel. Vitamin B and folic acid are essential to withstand as your body cannot generate them, and they are borrowed to stave off serious birth deformities. Calcium and vitamins can also be accepted into the contour of fruits and vegetables, but if you are not endorsing a good portion of fruits and salad, then it's better to take pills.

You are expected to be sensible that all sorts of vitamins are not integral in this phase. Vitamin A, D

& C should not be obtained during gestation as they can implicate the antenatal physique.

Here is further a list of sustenance that should not be ratified in the initial trimester, and you must avoid catching them.

Liver

It is malignant to the fetus if brought in high proportion because it comprises very drastic vitamin A

High Protein foods

Foods like raw or grilled egg, chicken, fish, lobster, etc. can be assumed in a very short percentage if necessary; regular intake may let your pregnancy in disorders because your unborn's body hierarchy is fragile and the body organs have the spare threat of disruption in the starting level.

Yeast and Pasteurized Milk

Food and confectionery entities that are given the rise of yeast are similarly not advised to be taken in these days; also, pasteurized milk and cheese are dangerous as they include bacteria and may cause upheaval. Other than that, you should stay away from unhygienic fast food and long term frozen items.

Synthetic sweeteners

The synthetic sweeteners which enclose saccharin and sodium cyclamate are not a fair inkling in these days, as well as avoid overuse of caffeine input because it may steer to the miscarriage or become risky for the arriving one. If you are a caffeine addict and could not cut it off totally, then you can use 2-3 cups per day.

Herbal Remedies

It might occur that the senior ladies in your family, relatives, or in neighborhoods tell some self remedies contemplating with your condition. Remember, appreciate their intention but do not rigorously pursue those instructions as they do not realize what your medical crisis really subsists, so avoid manipulating damn treatments.

Warning ⊘

Drugs, smoking, or alcohol is strictly prohibited in the whole duration, so don't bother yourself in seizing this nonsense.

Forthwith, glimpse the list of the diet which is apt for the mother in these days

Protein Intake

Yearn to accept protein on a regular rationale as they are the skyscraper for the body, and they can support the neonatal physique to be equipped competently.

Precautions:

Saturate a restricted percentage of high protein at the onset; afterward, you are free to use them.

Fatty Acids

Food gadgets that comprise fatty acids and omega 3 are positive for the baby's brain, so undertake a regular fraction of this nutrition.

Iron

Green vegetables are advantageous to generate iron in your body and erect hemoglobin status; they are effective to use in the meal; it will lift your blood level and fulfill the iron deficiency.

Milk and Yogurt

Milk is the perfect source of health. It does not merely furnish calcium and proteins to your body; also, it will be constructive to assemble your child's bones. Try taking milk and yogurt in a sufficient dose.

Fiber

Fiber, likewise, should be the greatly occupied portion for infusion, as it facilitates your food to digest and also make a strong body stake. Try using wheat, barley, and other fiber-enriched food and fruits

Water

For satisfactory digestion, upgrade in blood level, and deterred dehydration, you must carry a good volume of liquid, including water, juices, and herbal teas, which are free from caffeine.

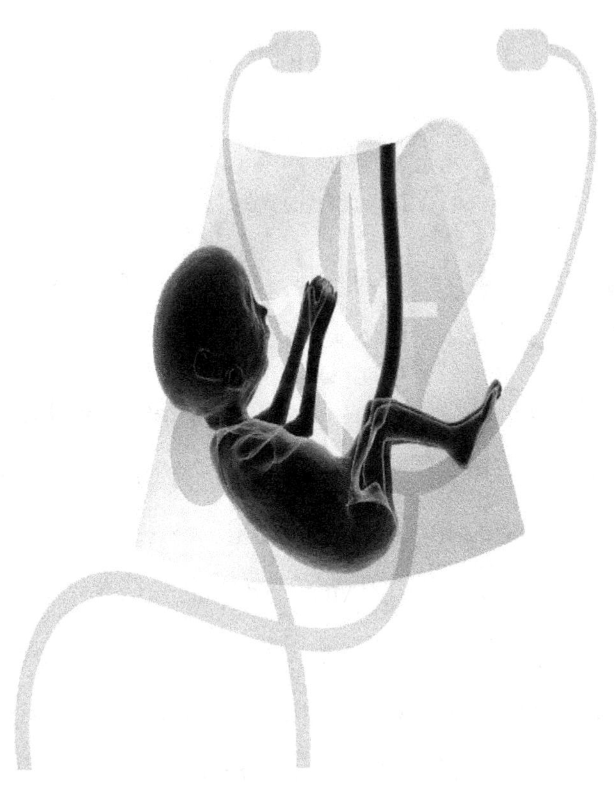

CHAPTER 2
2ND TRIMESTER, THE SAFEST DURATION

Welcome to your 2nd trimester!

Becoming a mother is an innate art, which is refined over time with experience!

This trimester starts from the 13th week of pregnancy and lasts till the 27th week. Your biological disposition becomes more stable in this stage, and now momentum to shift towards varied alterations in your body occurs. Practically, your earlier issues have departed to resolve in this, nausea, drowsiness, breathing difficulty, heartbeat problems, etc. all are receded now, and you feel yourself a bit energetic.

In 2nd trimester you feel better and energetic, now bring out time from your formal rituals and begin some fresh quirks which lend you pleasure and render your moments more remarkable. You can browse a list of baby and baba captions and select a beautiful name. Take a diary and prepare some plans regarding the recent change in your life. You can manuscript the pains and glows you feel in the whole pregnancy quest, inscribe your feelings for possessing a spirit in your belly, write each and everything you wish to do for the new guest. Write how much affectionate you are these days. You can also design in your diary that how you would organize the baby room, cot, or bedside so that when the time came, you are prepared to welcome the baby guest. Write it and keep with great compassion in your vault and when your baby comes to be of 7 or 8, show it to demonstrate your love to him/her.

What wonderful moments would those be!

If you are good at weaving or knitting, choose an outfit and formulate an elegant unisex layout in your complimentary moments to express love to your baby. Aim to deplete your leisure space in beautiful pastimes, visit natural locations, do slight gardening, see flowers and trees, scroll beautiful baby shots. Aloft, depart vigorous energies to earn your time beneficial to your health.

Interesting Fact:

Gawking beauty and nature in between pregnancy bring about your child pretty. Surviving merrily throughout pregnancy, makes your child innocent and soft tempered in real life.

Heavier Belly

You will experience some different occurrences this time; the most notable is the stretch on your gut.

As your baby gains weight, it will make your tummy heavier, your belly and breast size start heightening, and all this will make you apprehensive throughout, but you are required to take vigilance of your gestures and postures.

This is the time when you have to become open-eyed because a single unpredictable act can compel you in trouble. Be meticulous in changing your posture; if you are standing and want to sit down or lay down, you don't have to speed up or do not move in a hurry. Similarly, if you are lying on a bed and need to stand up, then move your body in a slow manner. As your midsection is going heftier day by day, do not keep standing unnecessarily, it will make you tired. When you walk, the burden of belly implicates your legs as well, and you can feel chronic pain in your feet and leg. Massage on your legs with coconut oil at night to have a good sleep.

Hungry all the time!

This is the period when you suffer from hunger double than normal, and it's beneficial for you to eat anything healthy right then because now you are not alone to consume the nutrition of your diet. Here your innocent baby is completely developed and needs ample food to accumulate and nourish so, what you eat normally is transferred to your baby as well, and that's why you feel hungry again and again. You may grab alternates in the form of snacks or salad in the day time, but if its night, do not take anything raw or deep-fried, it can cause heartburn or stomach disorder, so try fruits or bread at night. Restrain it in your intellect, 2nd trimester is the period when the baby craves more nutrition than further lengths, so do not keep your baby hungry at this time, whether you don't like to eat miscellaneously but eat for your child.

Interesting fact:

The babies who frequently stay ravenous in the mother's womb will reap the addiction of sucking their thumb in childhood.

As your belly expand, your breast size will also gain in a respective manner, to feel comfortable, and to stop the proliferation of the breast in an awkward way, you should use a comfortable air bra to remain at ease.

Now let's move to the sweep in body organs, especially in your belly. As the paunch is growing wider day by day, your skin snags tighter, which produces nuzzle massively.

Keep calm!

The biggest misstep done for the first time is often women enjoyably knead frequently on the whole tummy, and it results horribly. Your entire portion filled with stretch marks looks ugly. So when you feel stinging, stab to avoid maximum and if you are highly humiliated with it, then take a soft piece of cloth and rub it slowly and gently on the part; it makes you feel soft, and you will stave off from outrageous marks after delivering the baby.

Pregnancy Marks

Another aspect that offends women are the brown and grey spots on your body parts, including neck, the downside of your breast, abdomen, underarms, and under thighs, but here no need to worry about it because they are temporary patches and will wipe out after 2-3 months of labor. So, no need to sense awkward when discerning these spots, they are just due to the hormonal adaptation in your body. There may be some freckles on your face, especially on cheeks, nose, and chin. Be alert! This is the sign of iron deficiency in the body, and it especially increases after handing out birth due to excessive bleeding in case you go to scissor. If you start beholding freckles on your face, you should intake a sufficient quantity of iron after concerning the doctor.

Nasal Bleeding

Another serious issue is the nasal sensitivity during pregnancy. As your blood and hormonal level are boosted in these days, the mucous membrane becomes sensitive, sometimes due to a little gust or sneeze it started bleeding. It is recommended to you, when a visit to a doctor, you must inquire about the nasal bleeding, or you can use saline drops for the relief of nasal congestion.

Your gums and tissues become soft and sensitive; using a hard toothbrush may induce bleeding while flossing, so the smarter route is to use a softer toothbrush to impede your gums from bleeding and surging.

Discharge from Vagina

In this period, most women have a clammy and sticky vaginal discharge, which is not a serious problem; it is often normal, but if you feel pain in this discharge or it differs its color, or it causes smelly or sticky liquid then you must contact your doctor. Sometimes, due to the slight intake of water, your body is dehydrated, you can undergo an infection in urine bladder and feel difficulty in urinating. It can be treated by increasing aqueous quantity in the body, but if you feel smell or pain while passing urine, then it is not normally treated. You require medical assistance immediately. Otherwise, it will cause a serious kidney infection.

Monitor Baby

Now the time comes when your baby's weight and size are examined by your medical assistant, and your prenatal appointments become crucial to be done on time. When you head for a doctor, you would be asked for an ultrasound to see the baby's existing condition, the weight, size, and complete structure. Your recent hemoglobin will be reviewed through blood specimens, and some other tests will be done to evaluate each and every aspect regarding you and your baby. The fundal height will be checked by measuring the size of the uterus to investigate the chances of delivery. Some other screenings will be done, and you are advised to do a minor and sluggish walk in the 6th month. This juncture, you should improve your function level because the natural delivery attempts become intense when the mother maintained mobilizing in the second half of pregnancy. Try to do household chores yourself and make your rest time a bit shorter, but it doesn't mean to stress out with overworked make yourself much tired.

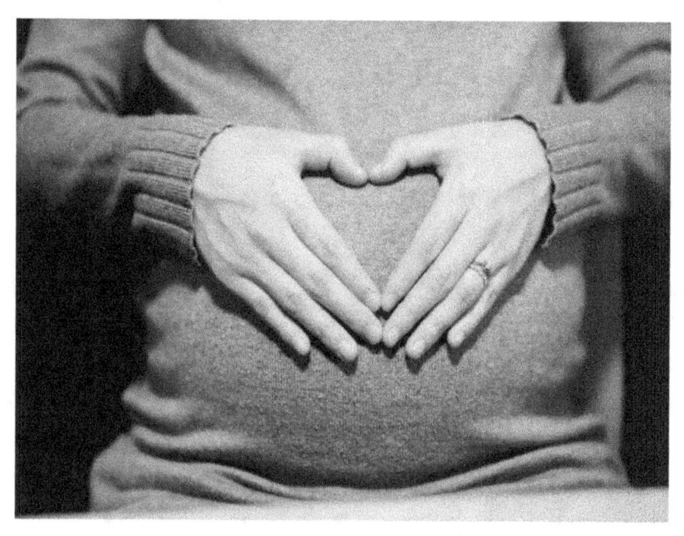

CHAPTER 3
FINAL STEP, THE THIRD TRIMESTER

How to get ready for child birth's drive to the third and the last trimester, which begins from 28th week and terminates when the baby comes into your lap. The time came when you have a dual responsibility, residing your own growths monitoring and the baby's each and every movement. Your physical condition is making you bulkier, and your belly is running wider and heavier, your buttocks are looking fluffed. All these physical changes are the sign of a healthy baby and also exhibit that everything is going pretty good, but it never means to be easy because it's the 7th month, the most critical for the baby. Now your baby has fully grown, all his organs are transforming in their original shape and size. However, the limbs are completely structured but still need to accumulate more, so be ready to fetch a larger bag with your belly. If you contemplate that there is no more room to expand your belly, then you are wrong, just wait and watch how fatty and wider you are going to be and how rapidly your baby is showing you the new existence. All of the time you will think

Huh! How much time remains to carry it more???

Some experts say:

The seventh month is very critical for the baby to be birthed, and the 8th month is critical for the mother to give birth.

Be obvious; you don't retain to go for any careless effort which can dominate you or your baby in any complication. Follow your doctor's advice in every aspect. Do not hide a single point of information regarding you and your baby to the doctor even if you forgot to implore in your visit, then make a phone call and acquaint the doctor to make sure if it is not anything serious. In this duration, your appointments will be more frequent, and you feel many changes and developments right then. These changes include the following factors of baby growth:

Your Baby's Size

Now your baby has completely developed, and his size and weight will be greater than the last trimester.

Approximate height: up to 20-22 inches

Approximate weight: up to 7-9 pounds

As the size increases, the uterus becomes congested for baby to survive, and so he starts kicking his leg to tell you.'

"I need more space, mama; please help!"

How silly!

Let's talk about the additional features which are now holding slot in the fetus.

Nervous System

This time the baby's brain has fully developed, and he concedes brandishing his brain and begins using dandy techniques as he thinks, moves his organs with the correspondence of brain, blinks his lashes, and regulates his body temperature.

Sense Organs Respond

After the 30th week, the five senses are ready to think, touch, see, smell, and taste. The young one tastes whatever you eat, listens to your whispers and music, touches the walls of his or her provisional home.

How do you think your baby knows the feel of you?

Skeleton

Though the whole skeleton was prepared ahead, it was made of cartilage, and now it is transporting into soft bones with the help of c calcium, and this calcium is draining to him from your body. Please take calcium filled pills and food which has natural calcium, take egg and milk, fish, etc. You can also use dry nuts in a score of 2 or 3 daily.

Hairs and Nails

In the 8th month of pregnancy, the baby's hairs and Nails develop appropriately, and you might feel stomach simmering due to the baby hairs that touch to the stomach's outer walls. Don't search for its cure because it is natural. The soft skin over the fingertips becomes a bit hard nails, and in the 9th month, the baby sheds his waxy coating outside, which is called vernix. Vernix helps prevent touching water bag fluid from touching the baby's skin.

Due to the last trimester, you also got some fingertips and pass through some aches and pains in which the most common are:

Backache

As your belly gains weight ratifying through days, you start feeling the ache in your back, which is due to the heavy abdomen, and also your bones' joints are lore loosened, but you have to carry your body with this pain till the last of D-day. You just stay calm!

Pain in the Abdomen

Just like back, your abdomen is also carrying some slack and undergoing pain; you should expect some rest after performing stints so that your abdomen gets relief. You don't have any other nice option.

Leg Pain

During your household chores or your job, you will suffer a tiresome pain or cramps in legs, which is discomforting your snooze as well. No matter how bad it is, No pain killers! Just use some lighter viscose oil to massage your legs.

Hemorrhoids and Varicose Veins

As your body is pumping additional blood, you will detect some bluish and purple veins chartered in the downside of your body; don't panic! They will vanish after your delivery.

Heartburn

Although your belly has tried to make enough room inside still, it needs more leeway. That's why it pushes your stomach up the side, which makes you feel heartburning and a slightly bitter taste in your throat. All of it is systematic, but if it is really bothering you, then ask your doctor to give a better suggestion.

Marks on Your Belly

Due to extra growth, your belly membrane is spanned and leaves some marks and smudges on your belly. Apply a moisturizer or a belly oil gently and wait for some months after delivering the baby. If they do not vanish, then use anti-marks cream with the consultation of a doctor.

Urinary Disturbance

Ow shit! What to do?

Having a slight leaking of urine due to a little sneeze or pee makes your sitting surroundings wet all the time. The baby's head lies on your bladder and makes it almost ready to flow. Keep any cotton swab to sit on.

Breast Leaking

The last days are near, and your breast is ready to feed, you may feel a little milky utterance.

Hungry Stomach

This time you can be filtering your fridge and kitchen cupboards to have something to eat. Take healthy food to keep yourself active, nap for a while in day time must be active throughout.

Over Bulk Body

When you see in the mirror, you will find a giant creature. Most of the body parts grow wider and larger that time and somebody parts might look swell. Don't be afraid of your widespread condition. It's just temporary and will re-size after the time.

Braxton Hicks Contraction

Are you feeling some pains and compressions?

It means your body is showing you pre-labor pains. Get ready for the final trial.

To-do list

You need to schedule many stints and jobs this trimester as your time of d-date is closer. However, your medical appointments are held to be earlier, and you are under complete observation of your doctor.

Mobility of the fetus

Time to be vigilant!

Now you have to monitor your child's movement and kicking. Measure them in a day, then the next day, and the third day. They shouldn't be equal all the days, but doing so makes you alert for any inconvenience movement all around so you can consult your GYN as early as possible.

Monitor Your Weight

In the introductory of the 7th month, your weight will constantly increase till the half of trimester, and afterward, it will decline 1-2 pounds typically. Keep watching your weight to get acknowledged if it is galloping on the right track. If you feel turmoil in progressing or relinquishing weight, go for medical assistance.

Keep Moving

Keep yourself mobilized throughout this term to make your d-procedure satisfactory. Do your households, go for a stroll and retain changing positions maximum of the time.

Scrutinize the Symptoms

As the fatal time is dispatching, you are going through various entities, which are the sign of coming closer to the labor day. These are called pre-birth warnings. You begin enacting with pursuing these actions

Pinkish Liquid Discharge Through the Mucous Plug

Hence, a mucus stain of pinkish blood release in a speck will start by the end of the 36th week, which tells that labor time is proceeding adequately. This liquid is dumping from the core of your uterus.

Squeezing to Labor

Feel the vigor of the Braxton Hicks as they boost their intensity rather than abate.

Perception of Lightening

As the infant reached the 36th week, you start experiencing anxiety as it is plummeting in your pelvis.

Water Sac Leaking

This is a discretionary process. Virtually it distills on the hospital bed but might possible due to any abrupt activity in your stance; it comes to be leaking. Be extremely cautious in this circumstance and arrive at the hospital as soon as possible.

Pre-birth Regular Visiting Schedule to your **Gynecologist**

In this term, your medical assistance is most crucial. You should be asked from the consultant to visit within a month, bi-monthly, and then weekly in respective order. You are instructed for several new analyses entailing

- Recent hemoglobin status

- GTT (Glucose testing treatment)

- Protein Level (if necessary)

You may be going through a physical checkup, including the innermost inspection of your cervix, to confirm the existing predicament, whether it began opening or not. If there is any complication assumption occurs, then your doctor will let you for the no-pressure test to make sure your trial.

You are requested to fill the birth form, which will be attached after in your biophysical profile that is made in your 1st visit of the initial trimester. It will assist the doctor further during your labor procedure.

In the expected last week of pregnancy, you are again done with an ultrasound to see the lying position of fetus, existence vein accessory (umbilical cord), the head size of the infant and etc.

Educate yourself about the labor facets

Being an early learner is good for this purpose, so while routine checkups consult your specialist about the probabilities of prematurity, strong and metamorphic childbirth also substantiate the warnings of labor pain

How to get ready for Childbirth

Brainstorm for the Final Decision Regarding Birth

The time is on the head to disseminate your way of labor to the doctor. You should know it before the time so that you can mentally prepare yourself for the upcoming phase.

Communicate! If you want to medicate for the birth suffering or going for the biological labor process, which doesn't possess impediments, whether you caught up with the medical birthplace on time or you birth the baby in your washroom etc. Although whatever you plan doesn't definitely proceed in the future as giving birth is a natural function, we can only organize it to keep off any discomfort or obstacle.

Sometimes, everything whacks as nicely as we attempt, and some distinct moments condition changes a handful. So, register a plan B too that can be accomplished if required, and you can not be terrified this way.

Labour Pain

This is a process for giving birth to a baby with natural pain; it is not of the same kind for all women. Some feel the severe contraction on uterus muscles and cervix; some feel pain and twitches as of menstrual cycle; likewise, some feel a heavy pressure on their urine tract. Hence it depends on the woman's physique and the way of pregnancy you pass through. In the US, there is a familiar Lamaze training that is given to their mothers to know the way of control that pain psychologically.

If you are nervous or in fear of birth pain, you may consult a specialist to take childbirth classes to get the confidence to relax on the labor bed.

Breast Feeding Awareness

Get ready to feed your new bud. Even though you are not used to breastfeeding, it's not a big deal.

You are under the strict observation

Remember one quirk, as you cross the 36th week, you can experience a force inside for pushing the baby out at any day between 37th to 40th week. Maybe you have to arrive hospital in an emergency situation, or you have the opportunity to admit a little before labor time. If you are advised for additional blood, arrange it before the time.

As you get the final date to be admitted to the hospital, start assembling the post-birth utilities. Pack your bag with integral commodities. Your bag includes:

- Baby costumes

- Baby wrap sheet

- Feeding bottle

- Towel

- Cotton

- Diapers pack

Did you forget the family care?

Your assignments have not ended; still, you yearn some endurance to plop it on other components skillfully.

Monetary Planning

Fold up your sleeves to increase your budget because you are going to have one more lovely life in your home. Make a new list of your home outlays comprising new one's requisites preliminary, synopsize their tariff, and see if you are prosperous with it financially or you anticipate to re-arrange in other moods.

Outline Your Baby Room

Including all stuff desired for your tot, maintain a vast spectrum of apparels, comforts, pampers and diapers, cotton swabs, pacifiers, etc. Jot down a welcome message to your newborn, stick on the baby bed and add some soft and beautiful hangings upwards the baby cot. Picture the room with beauty and nature. Paste lovely baby portrayals.

Don't forget your family

If you are the just matron in your house, then you prefer to refrigerate some supplementary dishes and cuisine to look after your folk in the busy baby domain after birth. Embark to tidy up all the surpluses in your home before getting on admitting because you don't know how many days you need to come out to a regular formality.

Good News

Conclusive eternity has come

As you feel the severe pain and pressure downwards to the abdomen, don't waste time, carry the bag and move to the hospital with your life partner. In case your partner is not available, immediately call him or leave a message, hire a cab and way towards the hospital.

Now good luck and have a safe journey!

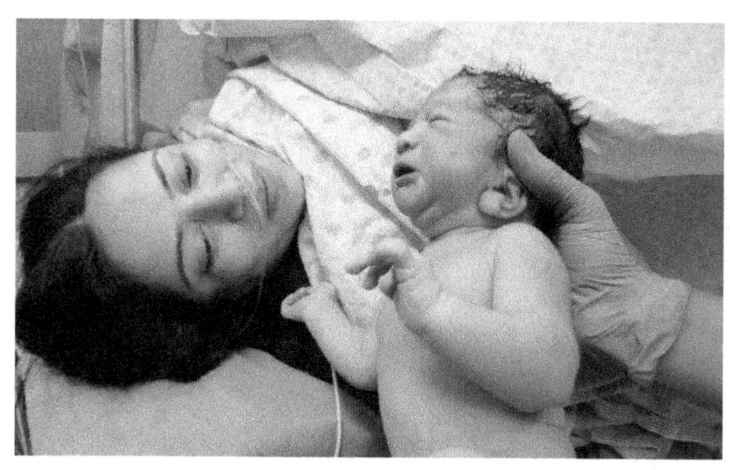

CHAPTER 4

BABY ARRIVAL. WELCOME HOME

Good-Bye to Labour

Welcome, Home, Baby!

Congratulations!

What a lovely gift you got after a long voyage

Now what to expect after childbirth?

Giving birth to a baby is tough, I understand, but did you guess you had succeeded the major obligation? Now you are linked in the new twist for the whole existence. As you know, mother's lap is the early institution for a child, so be comprehensive; your every stir will reproduce in your baby. Let him learn a good way of feeding first.

How do you think the baby should feed?

There is no particularly decided way to feed the baby; it's up to you; the way you feel comfortable, you can choose. Be careful; your posture should be productive for the baby latch. As the baby grows, feeding demands also change. Here are some useful feeding tips you can follow while feeding

Tips to be followed after your nine months

Use soft couches, cushions, or side pillows while lying for feeding so that you get ease during feed time.

Try best to be supportive for baby while feeding; do not let him bend for sucking.

Teach him proper latch. It will be useful for both mom and kid. Keep in your sanity. The way you start feeding will evolve permanently, so check your manner at the start. When the baby is not latching properly or if he does not suck in the right way, he might remain hungry or get habitual of sucking more and more.

Before starting feed, place your necessary stuff around your approach, especially wipes or tissue boxes, pieces of the towel, mobile phone, water bottle, television remote, a pack of chips, etc.

Maintain care of the baby but put up with some smart policies which make your life not so tangled; also, it impacts good habits on the baby.

Why make him habitual of limited attention?

Baby in your capes for the endless is not a good sensation. You have a lot of stations where to exhibit your love to him; do not pamper. Here are some tips for you to carry your baby the whole day.

Ready your food before time

Newborns feed in every couple of hours; you don't possess plenty of time in between, so strive to prepare your food before time. If you don't commit to it, you will persist hungrily and your baby then too due to scarcity of lactation.

Don't let your baby sleep while latching

Poke the baby ears slightly while feeding to render baby awake; this is because, if the baby slumbered between feed, the milk drops can linger in the feeding tube and stimulate siege of breath. After feeding, take him into your arms and pat slowly on the back so that air comes out, and he will sleep with ease.

Avoid baby sleeping in your arms.

Keep your baby in your arms or in a side lap just when you are free, or if he is crying, oppositely, don't let him in your hands each and every time. This habit makes baby and you both uncomfortable. Settle it in your mind that you are the reason to make him irritated. First, you carry him in your love; afterward, it's difficult to change his habit.

Monitor baby's signals

Babies cry! Yes, they do.

But what's the reason?

Not every time your baby cries for hunger, there

are several reasons. Find reasons, keep ears on their sound. You will discover that he cries out in varied sounds. Hungry baby screams impatiently and non stop while the wet diaper's sound has boisterous determination. When the baby gets bored with the quilt and wants an outside round, he makes noisy creaks only; don't weep with tears. So be careful, do not lay down for feed every time.

Don't be monotonous

Some mothers want their baby with them only; I know you love your baby a lot, and you are the supreme trustworthy person to him. Still, I suggest you make him a bit habitual of others, barely to your family partners do not share this strategy with outsiders. Let the baby play with the father to expand the kid's company.

Baby Sleep

Although it's old but very effective, sing a lullaby in a soft and gentle voice to make your baby's eyes shut, you can see the light of calm on his face. For delivering your baby a warm sleep, roll his sides with baby comforts after leaving him in a cot or baby mat.

Don't Let Diaper be wet

Leaving the wet diapers for long durations results badly. Baby skin is very delicate and cannot tolerate urinary enzymes and acids on the skin just for 10 minutes. It swells and produces rash skin, which upholds reddish crust. Check the diaper possibly in half-hour, respectively.

Baby massage and bath

Now it's time to understand giving bath to a baby; you could bath your baby after the shedding of the umbilical cord, but before providing him a bath, first take a good quality baby oil, as baby skin is the softest thing of all. Gently massage on the whole body afterward give a lukewarm bath to him.

Careful

Apply baby soap for a bath as beauty foams have chemical risks inside.

Never rinse your baby's face with a hand shower or a mug full of water; it will cause sniffing destruction. Always wet it from your handful of water, apply a little soap, and repeat to clean the face again.

Always use a baby bath seat or baby tub for giving a bath

Never leave your baby wet for a long time.

Apply baby moisturizer and baby powder after a bath. Do not sprinkle the baby powder directly on the face or other organs.

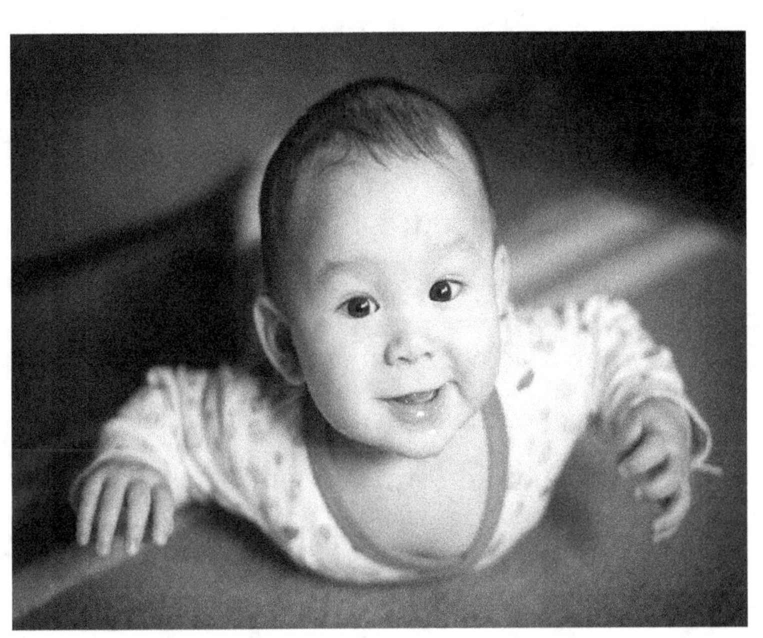

CHAPTER 5
TIPS TO FOLLOW AFTER NINE MONTHS

Postpartum, body and fitness care

Let's buzz on some physical aptitude.

When I was pregnant, I literally stopped seeing the mirror.

Oops! How horrible I looked. I planned many articles that could be done after my childbirth. My near women ensured me to confide some remedies, herbal extracts, and what not! Making my expanded figure in shape. I was excited, after birth, I will come to stand in my previous body, but all my enthusiasm flew away when I listened through a doctor to wait some more.

Subsequently, the birth scars are frigid, and your body has been sensitively fragile. Avoid committing superfluous physical workouts right after birth, and wait till the right moment, and your consultant gives you a green signal.

I know you are tired of your physical outcome and want to become as smart and gorgeous as you were. Not a big deal!

Here is a list of post-pregnancy recommendations, follow it, and fit your pre-baby figure. You might need a little more job to fulfill your body desire. Come out of your bedtime forfeiture. Do mental webbing for your after birth exercises.

Complete your Menstrual Cycle

Straight after birth, you will pass through extended bleeding, which is extremely vital to release. This blood is certainly replenished with junk organisms that were lingering in your body since the beginning of gestation. Occasionally, the bleeding quits in a short interval, and while serving any waits, it commences releasing again. This indicates that your uterus fences are sensitive and can be resulted in any injury or complication, so wait until your whole cycle is finalized, and meanwhile, your body gets to heal.

Instigate Your Postpartum in a Slow Manner

In my personal opinion, you should stay for a month or a half of it to begin toiling out if you have passed with the normal delivery. In the trial of a C-section, the scenario is totally different; you must wait for your next afterbirth checkup. Your uterus requires healing, and I think you may not want to mess your abdomen portion. Take your medicines on time, do rest and jerk your footsteps in a stagnant and soft manner. When you get sick off from rest and sleep, you can take a lukewarm water bath, hang outside and try a little trek of 4-5 minutes. Monitor your physical condition with this walk if you feel ease and don't want any urgent outcome then continue for a daily walk with steady increments. Remember, don't walk with your baby in your lap and do not exert force in trolling the baby. It's not a reasonable action for your personal health.

Tight up your joints

During the post-partum trip, the hormonal imbalance loses your hookups, and bones become to be ligamentous. They do not last right after delivery; almost they require more than 20 weeks. Your pelvis is also widened a bit, so prefer simple and minor influence efforts in postpartum exercises.

Pelvic Floor Muscles

During the whole pregnant journey, your pelvic suffers the most, carrying a continuous weight on it, and exerting a heavy push force while giving birth makes it vulnerable and uncomfortable. To strengthen your pelvic floor, you can start kegel exercise for the time being.

Kegel Exercise

Pass out urine and lie down straight with folding legs

Pull taut inside your pelvic floor in the way that muscles tight underside

Wait for 5 seconds with rigid holding

Relax the muscles for the exact duration

Repeat 10-15 turns

It can be attained in the morning, afternoon, and evening as per your solace.

Other than these, mothers can try:

- Lower burden activity

- Swimming

- Warm-up aerobics

- Yoga

- Walk

You can go through the great consequence of exercise by testing yourself in these light exercising days. If you feel any discomfort or random bleeding until the 12 weeks of birth, then consult your doctor and get more awareness about your health aspects. Do not let your time with easy go, always be cautious of your health as you are the main person to run a family.

Breastfeeding "A good opportunity."

If your infant is on Mother feed, then no need to upset more about your body's extra bulk because the more your baby will feed, your body size will shrink. This is the excess sap which you have taken in your pregnant duration and was reserved in your body, and it also surmised for looking intensified.

Improve your Water Intake

It is essential, especially for breastfeeding moms, to gulp an abundance of water because you need to stay hydrated throughout your feeding period. It will help to nourish your baby's stomach as well; it fulfills your hydration desire. Keep a boiled water container with you while going outside.

Don't get under sleep for a long time

It's almost vivid that moms get under rest after carrying a baby. I know there are tons of chores to conduct, and a to-do roster is in your mind for which you are in probe of a meager time. Nothing is terrific to your personal health. You stand on the 1st position in your family to handle in every facet, what will transpire if you get ill due to tiresome days? Afterward, you will not be able to do a single job, so be moderate and try to take a nap in a day time when your baby is sleeping.

Postpartum Depression

As the birth of a baby is an impetus effect of exertion of power during the labor time, this time, your whole body suffers from pain, and the vigor you applied to push the baby out makes your veins and muscles in grains. This results in a slight depression in your baby, and after birth, it looks a little bluish in complexion. The baby cries and gets sleep difficulty, but this blue effect will fade some after days.

Postpartum depression is another situation; it just not impact mood swings, nor is it your birth weakness. It is a disorder or complication of birth time. It considerably affects you and your baby. Not only them, but it also lasts for your whole family. Most of the time, mothers pass on a severe rotten condition at home due to postpartum depression, and they are not informed of the substantial issue. These depression signs are

- Lack of appetite

- Insomnia

- Falling energy level

- Fatigue

- Pessimism in mood

- Resentment

- Frustration

- Hopelessness

- Panic attacks

- Nightmares

- Isolation

- All times sleep

- Overeating

There are many other signs of depression. If you feel any of the signs (more than 3), you must visit the consultant as soon as possible and discuss your problem. Don't let it be ignored.

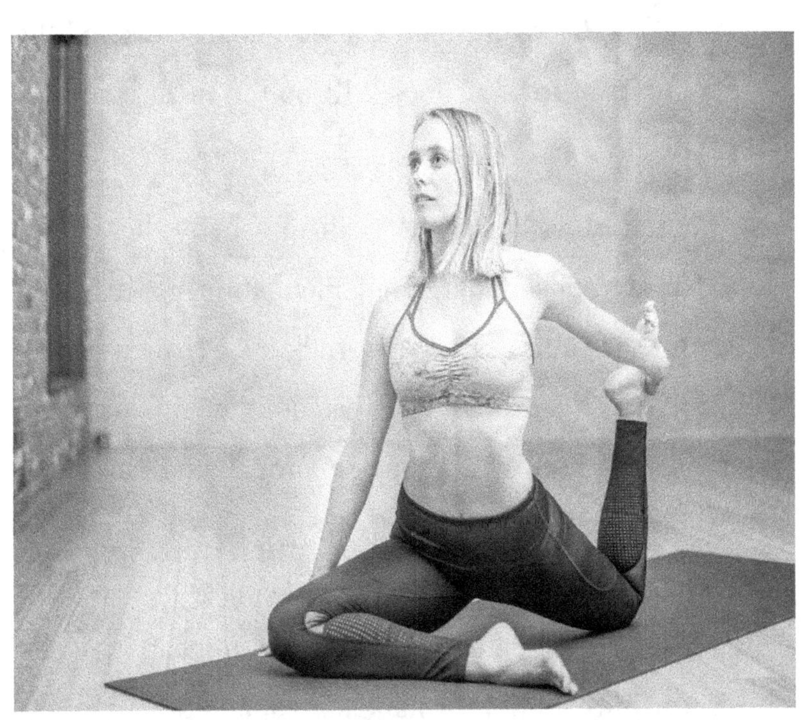

CONCLUSION

An indispensable ally with which you will discover that the next nine months and the following ones will be the most beautiful of your life!

When a mother gives birth to a baby, her bones and body cells undergo an incubation process and become as subtle as a newborn baby's. Now it's your prior duty to resume your previous health with the help of a good diet, proper exercise, and sufficient rest because, after birth, effects are very harmful to a woman's health. Your life is vital for you and your family. How could you carry a gear full of responsibilities if your hands are apathetic?

I hope reading this book will pull you out from the anxiety of being a super mom. Mom's duties are never won. You are employed as a mother for a lifetime permanent designation. Now it's up to you, how do you nourish your company of kids.

There are no fears for what is happening and will happen, but only deep emotions for love that is about to overwhelm you.

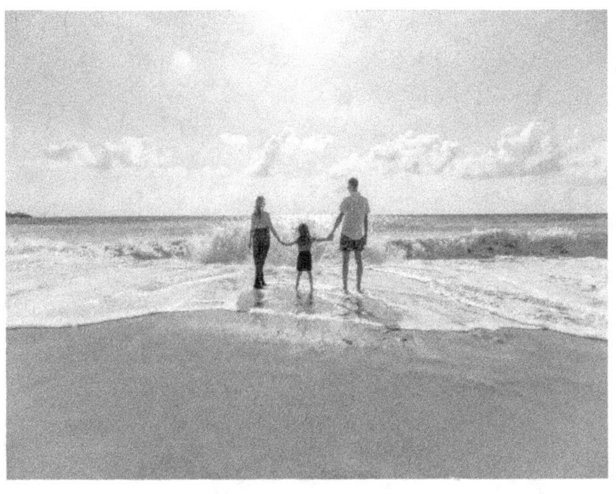

Good luck, moms!

Cristina Olsen